Managing Your Life

by Eating Right

Table Of Contents

Introduction

- 4 -

Are you eating just to whet your appetite or to satiate your taste buds? Or are you eating in order to take better control of your life?

In this eBook, we see how you can make your life much more optimal just by making sure that you eat right.

Chapter 1:

Why We Face Health Problems Today

Summary

The world is a lot unhealthier than it was two decades ago. A lot of this is attributed to the changed food habits of people.

Why We Face Health Problems Today

One generation ago, people would not dream of picking up whatever packet of junk food they could get at first in order to feed their faces. Today, we do that so very casually. "I am hungry" usually means "I want a hamburger or a frankfurter, probably with chips on the side and one cola." "Let's go out and party" means "Let's go out and booze till we can't stand up on our own and intersperse the drinks with as much synthetic-laden wannabe Chinese food that we can get." And, "I am on a diet" means "I am on a chemically driven pill which will kill my hunger and deprive my body of vitamins."

It is really no wonder that we are facing so many health problems today.

Our health is an indicator of what we eat. The sorry condition that we are living in is not an individual problem; it is a global problem. The world as a whole is eating wrong. Just check these facts out – 6 in every 10 persons in the US is overweight, and the number is going to be 8 in every 10 persons by the time we hit 2015. The US, the largest economy in the world, is spending close to $147 billion a year on healthcare due to various obesity-related issues. And this situation is true with most of the so-called developed nations of the world.

Now, if you just consider this one fact, think how much richer the US would have been if it didn't have to contend with this problem. The US reserves would have approximately $150 billion more each year which it could have used for developmental purposes. Probably, there would have been more schools and colleges (we know there is always a paucity of them), more research work being done, the lifestyle of people could be improved, and so much more. With that amount of money, the US could feed 3 third-world countries in Africa each year and rid them of all their food problems.

Are we really thinking about this? We aren't. Even as you are reading this eBook, you probably have a packet of Frito Lays on the side. Do you know that that packet, which is filling your stomach with some of the most toxic chemicals known to humans, could instead have fed an emaciated child in Rwanda?

But it's not just about being philanthropic. It's about ourselves too. Yes, we have to be selfish. With such alarming health figures, aren't we calling doom upon us? We are definitely not eating right. Whatever excess baggage that brings – obesity and the assorted health problems in its wake – we have to be prepared for it.

Chapter 2:

The Solution

Summary

Yes, there is cause for alarm. Our eating habits are plunging us into despair. But all is not lost, yet. We can still tighten our belts and look for solutions.

The Solution

We have erred horribly with our eating habits so far. Unless we take stock of the situation and take matters in our own hands, things are not going to improve.

The first thing is awareness. We have to learn what foods are right for us and what are not. We have to go back to school (not literally, of course) and understand what the nutrients are that your body really wants and in what measure. Then we have to work up a dietary regimen for ourselves and our family so that we eat healthier. We must cut down on all the foods that are harmful – the carbohydrates, the fats, the sugars, we don't really want them – and incorporate foods that can boost our health.

This does sound too preachy, I know. But that is the only respite we have got. If we keep munching on Oreos, we are never going to get better.

But there's hope. Hope lies in the fact that there are many foods out there that are just as tasty as those nasty junk foods but we don't yet know about them. These are the foods that we don't know about yet, we probably don't care for them or because we don't know how to prepare them, but a good health cookbook could help you in understanding various interesting ways to healthy cooking. Even with the same kind of diet you eat, you can conjure up some very delicious healthy dishes. Yes, it is all very much possible. You can modify your eating habits to a large extent, while at the same time taking care of your palate.

The fact is that the weight loss industry is responsible in a very significant way toward this downfall of the developed human race. They need to keep selling their Atkinses and Jenny Craigs and Zones and Medifasts and for that reason the media never tells you how we can actually take things in your own hands. They show us glitzy before-after pictures of a guy with a foot-long pannus and then the same guy with six pack abs and tell us that the diet made that possible.

But the fact is, if we were to take things in our own hands, we could very easily do that too, without needing to spend thousands of dollars on getting those diets. And what do we have to do? Two basic things:-
  ➢ Control what we eat.
  ➢ Indulge in physical exercise.

Now, is that too much to do? Don't we owe that to our body that has served us so well all these years? Don't we owe that to ourselves and our families?

Throughout this eBook we are going to see how we can eat right and generally modify our diet in order to improve our lives. And that we can do in a very significant manner.

Chapter 3:

What Is an Ideal Diet?

Summary

Eating right is essential. You need to know what the ideal diet is for that.

What Is an Ideal Diet?

Actually speaking, no one can put a finger on what an ideal diet exactly is. Now, if you were to ask someone what a healthy diet is, that could be easily answered. But to know about an ideal diet, you need to see the individual itself. Ideal diets are much related to the kind of lifestyle the person leads, their age, their gender, their level of physical activity during the day and even their geographical region and climate.

The first thing that must be answered here is the level of calories that any person must take. This, of course, varies from person to person, mainly depending on their level of physical activity. The following chart shows different kinds of people, characterized by various things, and the amount of calories that they need during the day, which would constitute an ideal diet for them.

People and Lifestyle	Required Calories per Day
Men leading a sedentary life	2,300
Men involved in high physical activity	3,200
Women leading a sedentary life	2,000
Women involved in high physical activity	2,500
Pregnant women	2,500
Lactating women	3,000
Infants up to a year-old	50, for each pound of body weight

Children between 1 and 10 years	1,000 – 2,000
Teenage boys	2,000 – 2,500
Teenage girls	1,500 – 2,000

Ideal diet depends from person to person, but there are some similarities that apply to every person:-

→ The diet should have enough carbohydrates, but not an excess of it. Excess of carbohydrates can cause buildup of glucose in the body.

→ Foods fried in oil must be minimally used. There should be just one serving of a fried food per day, if at all.

→ Green veggies must be a part of the meal. The general rule is that foods with better colors are more nutritious, though there are some exceptions both ways. i.e., There are foods with no colors that are nutritious (example, cabbage) and foods with colors that aren't (there's a whole long list of them).

→ Lean meats should be preferred. It is very harmful to have a meal that is laden with non-vegetarian foods but isn't balanced with vegetables.

→ Cooking should be just enough and must retain the natural flavors of the foods. Though spices make the foods taste better, they also destroy some nutrients and hence they should be used stingily.

→ Synthetic materials should be completely avoided.

Chapter 4:

Benefits of Eating Right

Summary

Here is all the motivation you would need to keep eating healthy.

Benefits of Eating Right

Let's directly plunge into the topic.

Makes You Healthier

We could write a whole compendium about the health benefits of eating right and still it wouldn't quite cover what benefits really exist. The most significant benefit is that you gain control over your weight. By eating right, you also make sure that your metabolic functions – most notably your immune system and your digestive system – keep working right. You are also protected from various chronic diseases, right from cardiovascular diseases like atherosclerosis and high blood pressure to diabetes.

More Money for You

Eating healthy means you spend a lot less. Your bills at the supermarkets reduce drastically and you don't plunge further into credit card debt if that is already a problem with you. Also, you save a big bundle on all the healthcare expenses you would need if any problem surfaces because of your food binging habits.

Less Toxic Foods in Your Body

Many foods today are toxic because of the synthetic chemicals present in them. When you are trying to eat right, you are much less likely to get these toxins into your body because one of the basic tenets of eating right is that you shouldn't eat anything that is synthetic. Also, when you eat less, you will also be able to reduce on vices such as smoking and alcoholism. A glass of beer is almost synonymous with a night out with the boys. When you eat less, you won't want the beer too. Similarly, you will not want that one (or more) mandatory smoke that you tend to have after every full meal.

More Active Lifestyle

When you eat better, you will find that you can do your work in a much better way. You can exercise more, travel more, play more, work more and thus make your life more productive. That sure beats being a fat slob and lounging around on the couch the whole day, doesn't it? You can also be more involved with your friends and family and that certainly enriches your life.

Better Social Life

Forget about feederism and fat fetishism, people who are overweight do not look appealing. There's a strong social taboo about weight on the wrong places of the human body. If you are trying to find a partner, your flab could literally come in the way. Not just that, people who cannot control their eating habits and hence their weight are looked down upon by society as being people who cannot control their basic urges. This kind of psychology does exist, though very few people will speak about it. When you eat right, you will find that such problems disappear.

Chapter 5:

Losing Weight by Eating Right

Summary

Most of you who have downloaded this eBook will want to read about this part. So here goes – how do you lose weight by eating right?

Losing Weight by Eating Right

You can easily find a lot of information about eating right to lose your weight. But there are some things that are more important than the food itself. Let us tackle those things first. Without these, your weight loss would be a wasted effort.

Motivation

No one can effectively lose their weight without the right motivation. You have to have something in mind as your goal; that is what keeps you determined. This goal could be the need to look better (read, slimmer), or to be healthier, or to be more physically active, anything. Then you have to set your mind upon this goal. It is this aim that you have to think about. When you are sure about where you want to reach, you are able to chalk out your path in a much better way.

Support and Encouragement

Though there are people who have lost weight all by themselves, things are made much simpler if they have family and friends to support them. They should keep encouraging them, not ridiculing them, and then the system works. There are people who have lost weight just because they can be more productive in their family life. This can be a very strong feeling and can work highly in losing weight.

It is also very effective if you can go on a weight loss program with someone else. Even a little competitive edge helps. In fact, competition can work nicely. There's nothing better than the need to show someone that you can do something.

The actual eating regimen comes later.

Now, don't get swayed by the various food fads that you see on the Internet. These are absolutely not necessary. What you need is your own determination and some effort in choosing the right foods.

It is best to prepare a complete health plan and stick with it. You will find one such health plan here:-
http://www.joyfullivingservices.com/idealdiet.html

If you are looking for a plan for a child, then here is a good resource:-
http://www.vegsource.com/attwood/stages.htm

These diets can work very well and you won't need a fad diet to help you. You can be your own fitness guru.

Chapter 6:

Eating Right Is Not the Only Thing

Summary

There are other things you need to lead a complete life. Merely eating right is not enough.

Eating Right Is Not the Only Thing

You must have heard time and again how important it is to supplement your dietary habits with various other healthy lifestyle aspects in order to enrich your life. Diet is one part of our lives – a very important part too – but it is not the only thing. Exercise is the first thing that comes to mind when we speak about a supplement to diet. We already know the great importance of physical exercise. If you are going to eat right but still you are going to stay a couch potato, then there's very little benefit that you are going to get out of your newly improved eating habits.

There are various other such things that we have to supplement with our right eating habits and exercise. Here is a list.

Positive Attitude

A person who is always optimistic and zestful about life is likely to do better in every walk of life. The positive attitude is a very important element of wellbeing.

Chapter 7:

Managing Food, Family and Friends

Summary

Sometimes, we feel we are neglecting our family and friends when we are trying to do something for ourselves. This is where the feeling of vanity steps in.

Managing Food, Family and Friends

A lot of people end up paying a lot more than they bargain for when they enter into a healthy eating program. These are the things I have heard:-

"I started a natural eating program for my kids at home, and now they hate me for it." – A housewife with three kids.

"Did I do something wrong? My husband thinks I am more obsessive about my waistline than I am about him." – A 20-year old wife.

"I just missed a party invitation because they thought I wouldn't want the temptation to come my way." – An office-going middle-aged male.

These things are very natural. We enter a dietary program and then such things happen. The first thing to overcome is the mockery of people around us. Yes, there are people who will mock you if you start a diet. But then, we must remember that there are many more people who will mock us if we don't go on a diet and keep piling up those pounds.

The second problem is that the person who is on a healthy eating routine will want other people around them to get into it too. Women will try to influence the other people in their family to eat healthier too, and men will try to do that when they are among their group of friends. Now, you have to realize one thing. Even you weren't onto this healthy eating plan until you got fully convinced about it. You did not start right away, did you? You took your time. It was only when realization dawned upon you that you have to take care of your health did you begin taking things more seriously. But now that you have started your healthy eating program, you should not expect others to get into it right away too. They will take their time, if at all they decide to keep eating health. Do your best in convincing them by explaining the health benefits they would get and all the other benefits they'll have when they start eating healthy. But don't start force-feeding them those sprouts yet.

One more thing is that people who are on a healthy eating program tend to make a much bigger deal of it than it actually is. They will want everyone to know what supreme food sacrifices they are making. They will tell everyone that they are skipping meals and eating only things that are considered healthy, etc. But this might actually put you outside some social circles. Like, your friends may not even call you the next time they are going to Taco Bell. Instead, the best approach would be to let your friends know that you do let your hair loose once in a while, which you must do really to avoid the stress. That way, they won't be much bothered about your eating habits.

Chapter 8:

Your Motivations for Eating Right

Summary

You need the right motivation for whatever you do, more so if you are trying to get into a difficult healthy eating program.

Your Motivations for Eating Right

It is difficult for most people to get into a healthy eating program. You have been eating all those fried foods and pumping all those cokes and beers for such a long time now that even thinking about giving them all up can be a nightmare. In fact, most people don't think about eating healthy because of this paranoia associated with dieting. They don't think they will be able to survive it. But, of course, you need not be so excruciating on yourself right from the start. Start slow, drop one type of food at a time. You don't necessarily have to stop everything you eat if you can reduce the quantity and frequency. Alternatively, you could eat healthy through the week and have a small feast for one of your weekend meals. These are some ways to get around the confinement of healthy eating, but even so people need motivation.

Always Keep a Goal in Mind

The stronger your goal is, the more motivated you will be. This goal could be anything – you want to look better before an upcoming social event, you want to feel better, you want to become more active and energetic, you want to do things that you cannot do because of your weight, you want to keep living a healthy life, or simply that you want to show a friend who ridiculed you! The important thing is that you have to keep this goal sternly in mind and then use it as your motivating factor.

Resolve that You Won't Give Up

If you make a resolution that you won't give up, you will find it harder to deviate from your healthy eating regimen. If possible, make this resolution in front of your family or friends or the colleagues at work. This helps because whenever you are tempted to eat something unhealthy, you will remember your resolution and will stop.

Pick Up a Difficult Hobby

You could try getting yourself interested in something that is difficult for you to do at the moment, but will become easier once your body is in better shape. Swimming and dancing are good choices. These activities can keep you much interested if you try them out once, but you will need to get in better shape to do them well. The fun part is that when you swim or dance, you are automatically losing weight!

Get a Partner

This is the best motivation you could get. Get someone else with a similar problem to start the program of healthy eating with you. The two of you will be great encouragers for each other. You could even compete against each other and check out who is doing better. This helps because you are not alone in this mission; you have company.

Chapter 9:

How Not to Become Obsessive about Eating Right

Summary

We must eat right, but to what extent? How far can we take this?

How Not to Become Obsessive about Eating Right

It is important to eat right, but it is also important not to become obsessive about it. That is when the problems begin.

Obsession about eating right could lead to several complications. You might get unduly stressed out several times. When you are stressed out, you release a hormone known as cortisol. This has an adverse effect on the body. Cortisol slows down the metabolic processes of the body and hence the weight problem gets much aggravated.

This is just one reason why you should not get obsessive about eating right. There is also the problem that you might be depriving your body of the required amount of nutrition by drastically reducing your food intake. You might not be getting the vitamins that your body needs to develop properly and that could lead you to problems with dietary deficiency diseases. Also, impaired nourishment may cause anorexia, a condition that can open up a whole Pandora's Box of health ailments.

Then there is the social aspect to consider. Wittingly or unwittingly, you might be tormenting other people with your food obsessions as we have seen earlier.

Hence, it is important that you don't carry your eating right habit so far that it becomes an obsession. You are doing this to manage your life, but don't let it control your life.

The best way is to treat yourself once in a while. Let yourself go on that one day of the week. Take your family along. This could be a Sunday dinner. This is the day your family knows you permit yourself to eat anything. Have a glorious meal that day, mostly as a reward for keeping up through the week. In fact, if you take this in the right spirit, every Sunday could be a sort of festival for you.

Don't stress yourself too much, and it won't become an obsession. There are several breathing and mind control exercises that you can use. Make your mind healthier along with your body. This is the best way to prohibit the stresses from ravaging your mental space. You can learn these exercises from the various fitness programs they show on television and also from several videos on places such as YouTube.

Chapter 10:

Eating Right and Managing Your Life

Summary

Eat right, live well.

Eating Right and Managing Your Life

When you eat right for a while, you will find that automatically things begin falling into place. Your life suddenly becomes much better and you see that you start gaining control of it. And all this happens because you have now taken control of your eating habits.

The most important thing is that you have to stay driven. Probably you started with an 'eat right' program because you had some extra pounds in your body. Through your constant efforts, you have now managed to overcome that situation. Your body is in much better shape now. But that doesn't mean you can start going on food binges now. You have to continue with your healthy eating regimen. Only then will you experience its true effects in managing your life.

If you stay on a healthy eating program for two months at a stretch, you will stay on it for life. That's a fact. Hence, it is just those two months that you have to stay focused. You will find that the benefits you get within those two months will keep you hooked onto the program forever.

Read books, watch videos, research on the Internet, find out situations and examples of people who have brought their lives under control by moderating their eating habits. You will find a lot of inspiration from these stories and will want to implement them in your life too.

So, stay on it. If you are looking at improving the way you manage physical tasks or want to improve your stamina or want to just shed some undesired weight, eating right is the way to go about it. You will be able to get all these benefits and, most importantly, you will be able to spend more quality time with your family and friends. This is what will really help in managing your life and making it more meaningful, if nothing else.

Conclusion

Managing your life is in your own hands. Eating right is one of the best ways to go about it.

You now know what that means to you.

Go ahead and chalk out a healthy eating program for yourself today.

All the best to you!!!